Revitalize Your Gut

50 Superfoods for Optimal Digestive Health and Healing

By

Charles L. Rivera

TABLE OF CONTENTS

Introduction

Are you ready to unlock the secret to a revitalized you? Welcome to "Revitalize Your Gut: 50 Superfoods for Optimal Digestive Health and Healing," a transformative journey that will ignite your passion for gut wellness and lead you to a life of vibrant health and happiness.

Picture a life free from the discomfort of digestive issues, where every meal brings joy and nourishment to your body and soul. In this emotional and empowering guide, you will embark on a deeply personal exploration of the incredible healing potential within your gut.

Your gut is more than just a digestive system; it's a powerhouse of vitality and well-being. "Revitalize Your Gut" reveals the extraordinary healing power of 50 superfoods, carefully curated to restore balance, promote optimal digestion, and unleash a renewed sense of vitality within you.

Prepare to be captivated by the stories behind each superfood, as you uncover the profound connection between gut health and your overall well-being. With each turn of the page, you'll be inspired to nourish your body with vibrant berries bursting with antioxidants, nutrient-packed greens that invigorate your senses, and wholesome grains that provide sustained energy and nourishment.

But this journey isn't just about food. It's about embracing a new way of life, one that honors and cherishes your gut. It's about reclaiming your power, making choices that fuel your body with love and compassion. It's about stepping into a future where you radiate vitality from the inside out.

Are you ready to embark on this transformative path to gut wellness? Open the pages of "Revitalize Your Gut" and let your journey begin. Your revitalized self awaits.

Chapter One

The Power of Superfoods

Superfoods have become the buzzword in the world of health and nutrition. These food items are packed with essential nutrients, vitamins, and minerals that help improve your overall health. Incorporating superfoods into your diet can help prevent chronic diseases, boost immunity, and promote weight loss.

One of the primary benefits of superfoods is their ability to enhance digestion. They contain high amounts of dietary fiber, which acts as a prebiotic, providing fuel for the beneficial bacteria in your gut.

A flourishing gut microbiome translates into improved nutrient absorption, reduced digestive issues, and a strengthened immune system.

Moreover, superfoods are known for their anti-inflammatory properties. Chronic inflammation in the gut can lead to various health issues. However, the powerful antioxidants and phytonutrients present in superfoods help combat inflammation, promoting a calmer and healthier gut environment.

Incorporating superfoods into your diet can bring a multitude of benefits, including increased energy levels, improved mood, and enhanced overall well-being.

These nutrient-rich foods support your body's natural detoxification processes, provide essential vitamins and minerals, and contribute to maintaining a healthy weight.

Chapter Two

Superfoods for Revitalizing the Gut

Fiber-Rich Foods

CHIA SEEDS

Description: Small seeds with a gel-like texture when soaked.

Nutritional Profile:

- High in fiber
- Omega-3 fatty acids
- Antioxidants.

Unique Benefits:

- Promote bowel regularity
- Support a healthy gut microbiome.

FLAXSEEDS

Description: Tiny seeds with a nutty flavor, often ground into a powder.

Nutritional Profile:

- Rich in fiber and
- lignans.

Unique Benefits:

- Aid digestion
- Reduce inflammation
- Support gut health.

OATS

Description: Whole grains commonly consumed as oatmeal or in baked goods.

Nutritional Profile:

- High in soluble fiber.

Unique Benefits:

- Act as a prebiotic
- Nourish beneficial gut bacteria
- Promote a healthy digestive system.

QUINOA

Description: Ancient grain with a nutty flavor, versatile in various dishes.

Nutritional Profile:

- Contains fiber and
- Essential amino acids.

Unique Benefits:

- Support a healthy gut
- provide essential nutrients for overall well-being.

BERRIES

Description: Colorful fruits such as blueberries, raspberries, and strawberries.

Nutritional Profile:

- Rich in fiber
- Antioxidants and
- Vitamins.

Unique Benefits:

- Protect the gut from oxidative stress
- Reduce inflammation
- Promote a healthy digestive system.

Fermented Foods

KIMCHI

Description: Traditional Korean dish made by fermenting vegetables with spices.

Nutritional Profile:

- Fermented vegetables rich in probiotics.

Unique Benefits:

- Promote gut health
- Enhance digestion
- Boost the immune system.

KEFIR

Description: Fermented milk drink with a tangy flavor and creamy consistency.

Nutritional Profile:

- Contains probiotics and
- Protein.

Unique Benefits:

- Provide beneficial gut bacteria
- Support a balanced gut microbiome.

SAUERKRAUT

Description: Fermented cabbage with a sour taste, used as a condiment.

Nutritional Profile:

- Packed with probiotics and
- Fiber.

Unique Benefits:

- Aid digestion
- Boost the immune system
- Promote gut healing.

YOGURT

Description: Dairy product made by fermenting milk with live bacteria cultures.

Nutritional Profile:

- Contains probiotics and
- Protein.

Unique Benefits:

- Maintain a healthy gut flora
- Support digestion.

KOMBUCHA

Description: Fermented tea beverage with a slightly effervescent quality.

Nutritional Profile:

- Contains probiotics and
- Beneficial organic acids.

Unique Benefits:

- Promote a balanced gut microbiome
- Support digestion
- Boost immune function.

Omega-3 Rich Foods

SALMON

Description: Fatty fish known for its pink flesh and rich flavor.

Nutritional Profile:

- High in omega-3 fatty acids and
- Protein.

Unique Benefits:

- Reduce gut inflammation
- Support a healthy gut environment.

WALNUTS

Description: Nut with a hard shell and wrinkled appearance.

Nutritional Profile:

- Rich in omega-3 fatty acids and
- Antioxidants.

Unique Benefits:

- Support gut health
- Reduce inflammation
- Improve gut barrier function.

HEMP SEEDS

Description: Seeds derived from the hemp plant, often used in seed form or oil.

Nutritional Profile:

- High in omega-3 fatty acids and
- Protein.

Unique Benefits:

- Reduce gut inflammation
- Support gut health.

DARK CHOCOLATE

Description: Rich and indulgent treat made from cocoa beans.

Nutritional Profile:

- Contains antioxidants and
- Flavonoids.

Unique Benefits:

- Reduce gut inflammation
- Support a healthy gut environment.

GREEN LEAFY VEGETABLES

Description: Nutrient-dense vegetables like spinach, kale, and Swiss chard.

Nutritional Profile:

- High in antioxidants
- Vitamins and
- Minerals.

Unique Benefits:

- Promote gut health
- Reduce inflammation
- Support a healthy gut microbiome.

TURMERIC

Description: Vibrant yellow spice commonly used in curry dishes.

Nutritional Profile:

- Contains curcumin
- A powerful antioxidant.

Unique Benefits:

- Reduce gut inflammation
- Support gut healing
- Promote overall digestive health.

GINGER

Description: Pungent and aromatic root commonly used as a spice and herbal remedy.

Nutritional Profile:

- Contains antioxidants and
- Anti-inflammatory compounds.

Unique Benefits:

- Soothe gastrointestinal discomfort
- Aid digestion
- Reduce inflammation in the gut.

TOMATOES

Description: Red and juicy fruits commonly used in various dishes.

Nutritional Profile:

- Rich in antioxidants and
- Vitamins.

Unique Benefits:

- Protect against gut inflammation
- Support overall digestive health.

GREEN TEA

Description: A refreshing beverage made from the leaves of Camellia sinensis.

Nutritional Profile:

- Contains antioxidants and
- Polyphenols.

Unique Benefits:

- Reduce gut inflammation
- Support gut healing, promote a healthy gut microbiome.

Probiotic Foods

GREEK YOGURT

Description: Thick and creamy yogurt with a higher protein content.

Nutritional Profile:

- Contains probiotics and
- Calcium.

Unique Benefits:

- Promote the growth of beneficial gut bacteria
- Support digestion.

TEMPEH

Description: Fermented soybean cake with a nutty flavor and firm texture.

Nutritional Profile:

- Rich in probiotics
- Protein, and
- Fiber.

Unique Benefits: Support a balanced gut microbiome, aid in nutrient absorption.

MISO

Description: Fermented soybean paste with a salty and savory taste.

Nutritional Profile:

- Contains probiotics and
- Essential amino acids.

Unique Benefits:

- Support gut health
- Strengthen the immune system.

PICKLES

Description: Cucumbers or other vegetables preserved in brine or vinegar.

Nutritional Profile:

- Contains probiotics and
- Antioxidants.

Unique Benefits:

- Promote a healthy gut flora
- Aid digestion.

FATTY FISH

Description: Fish like salmon, mackerel, and sardines rich in omega-3 fatty acids.

Nutritional Profile:

- High in omega-3 fatty acids and
- Protein.

Unique Benefits:

- Reduce gut inflammation
- Support gut health
- Protect against inflammatory bowel diseases.

LEAFY GREEN VEGETABLES

Description: Nutrient-dense vegetables like spinach, kale, and Swiss chard.

Nutritional Profile:

- Rich in antioxidants
- Vitamins, and
- Minerals.

Unique Benefits:

- Reduce gut inflammation
- Support a healthy gut microbiome
- Promote overall digestive health.

Prebiotic Foods

GARLIC

Description: A pungent and aromatic bulb widely used in cooking.

Nutritional Profile:

- Contains prebiotic fibers and
- Antioxidants.

Unique Benefits:

- Nourish beneficial gut bacteria
- Support gut health.

ONIONS

Description: Bulb vegetables with a strong flavor used in various cuisines.

Nutritional Profile:

- Rich in prebiotic fibers and
- Antioxidants.

Unique Benefits:

- Promote the growth of beneficial gut bacteria
- Support digestive health.

ASPARAGUS

Description: Green spears with a distinct flavor and tender texture.

Nutritional Profile:

- Contains prebiotic fibers
- Vitamins, and
- Minerals.

Unique Benefits:

- Enhance the growth of beneficial gut bacteria
- Support gut health.

JERUSALEM ARTICHOKE

Description: Edible tuber with a nutty and sweet taste.

Nutritional Profile:

- Rich in inulin
- A prebiotic fiber.

Unique Benefits:

- Feed beneficial gut bacteria
- Improve digestion
- Support a healthy gut microbiome.

BANANAS

Description: Soft and sweet fruit with a yellow peel.

Nutritional Profile:

- Contains prebiotic fibers
- Vitamins, and
- Minerals.

Unique Benefits:

- Stimulate the growth of beneficial gut bacteria
- Promote regular bowel movements.

Gut-Soothing Foods

ALOE VERA

Description: Succulent plant with gel-filled leaves used for its medicinal properties.

Nutritional Profile:

- Contains vitamin
- Minerals, and
- Antioxidants.

Unique Benefits:

- Soothe and heal the gut lining
- Reduce inflammation in the digestive tract.

BONE BROTH

Description: A nourishing broth made from simmering bones and connective tissues.

Nutritional Profile:

- Rich in collagen
- Amino acids, and
- Minerals.

Unique Benefits:

- Support gut integrity
- Reduce inflammation
- Aid in gut healing.

PEPPERMINT

Description: A fragrant herb often used for its refreshing flavor.

Nutritional Profile:

- Contains menthol and
- Antioxidants.

Unique Benefits:

- Soothe gastrointestinal discomfort
- Reduce bloating
- Improve digestion.

MARSHMALLOW ROOT

Description: Herb with soothing properties often used in herbal remedies.

Nutritional Profile:

- Contains mucilage
- Polysaccharides and
- Antioxidants.

Unique Benefits:

- Soothe the gut lining
- Reduce inflammation
- Support digestive health.

SLIPPERY ELM

Description: Herbal remedy derived from the inner bark of the slippery elm tree.

Nutritional Profile:

- Contains mucilage and
- Antioxidants.

Unique Benefits:

- Soothe and protect the digestive tract
- Support gut healing.

APPLE CIDER VINEGAR

Description: Fermented apple juice commonly used as a condiment or health tonic.

Nutritional Profile:

- Contains acetic acid and
- Antioxidants.

Unique Benefits:

- Support digestion
- Improve nutrient absorption
- Promote a healthy gut microbiome.

COCONUT OIL

Description: Edible oil derived from coconuts.

Nutritional Profile:

- Contains medium-chain triglycerides (MCTs).

Unique Benefits:

- Possess antimicrobial properties
- Support gut health.

POMEGRANATE

Description: Fruit with a vibrant red color and juicy arils.

Nutritional Profile:

- Rich in antioxidants and
- Vitamins.

Unique Benefits:

- Reduce gut inflammation
- Support a healthy gut microbiome.

These superfoods can help revitalize your gut by providing essential nutrients, promoting gut health, and supporting overall digestion.

Incorporating them into your diet can contribute to a healthier gut and improved well-being. Remember to enjoy them as part of a balanced and varied eating plan.

Simple and delicious recipe ideas that incorporate Gut superfood

BERRY CHIA PUDDING

- Combine 1 cup of Greek yogurt
- 2 tablespoons of chia seeds, and
- A handful of mixed berries.
- Mix well and let it sit in the refrigerator overnight.

In the morning, enjoy a creamy and nutritious chia pudding loaded with probiotics and antioxidants.

TURMERIC GINGER SMOOTHIE

- Blend 1 cup of unsweetened almond milk
- 1 frozen banana,
- 1 teaspoon of turmeric powder, and
- A small piece of fresh ginger.
- Add a palmful of spinach or kale for extra greens.

Enjoy a refreshing and anti-inflammatory smoothie that supports gut health and boosts your immune system.

QUINOA SALAD WITH ROASTED VEGETABLES

- Cook 1 cup of quinoa according to the package instructions and let it cool.
- Roast a variety of colorful vegetables such as bell peppers, zucchini, and cherry tomatoes.
- Toss the cooked quinoa with the roasted vegetables,
- Drizzle with olive oil and lemon juice, and
- Sprinkle with fresh herbs like parsley or basil.

This nutrient-packed salad is rich in fiber, antioxidants, and essential nutrients.

PROBIOTIC BOWL WITH KIMCHI

- Start with a base of cooked brown rice or quinoa.
- Top it with sautéed kale, sliced avocado, and a scoop of probiotic-rich kimchi.
- Add a soft-boiled egg or grilled tofu for a protein boost.
- Drizzle with a soy-ginger dressing for a flavorful and gut-healthy bowl.

SUPERFOOD TRAIL MIX ENERGY BARS

- In a food processor, blend together dates, almonds, pumpkin seeds, chia seeds, and a tablespoon of cacao powder.
- Compact the blend into a baking dish and chill until it solidifies.
- Cut into bars and enjoy these homemade energy bars packed with nuts, seeds, and antioxidants.

MISO-GLAZED SALMON

- Mix together 2 tablespoons of miso paste,
- 1 tablespoon of maple syrup, and
- 1 teaspoon of grated ginger.
- Brush the mixture over salmon fillets and bake at 400°F (200°C) for about 15-20 minutes.
- Serve the miso-glazed salmon with a side of steamed broccoli or roasted Brussels sprouts.

This dish is not only delicious but also provides omega-3 fatty acids and gut-supporting probiotics.

GUT-HEALING BONE BROTH SOUP

- Simmer bone broth with a mix of vegetables like carrots, celery, and onions.
- Add shredded chicken or tofu for added protein.
- Season with turmeric, ginger, and garlic for their anti-inflammatory properties.

Enjoy a comforting and nourishing soup that supports gut healing and overall wellness.

AVOCADO AND HEMP SEED TOAST

- Toast a slice of whole-grain bread.
- Spread mashed avocado on top and sprinkle with hemp seeds.
- Season with a pinch of sea salt and black pepper.

Enjoy a satisfying and nutrient-dense breakfast or snack that provides healthy fats, fiber, and plant-based protein.

SUPERFOOD STIR-FRY

- Heat a tablespoon of olive oil in a pan and add diced tofu or chicken.
- Stir-fry with a variety of colorful vegetables like bell peppers, broccoli, and snap peas.
- Add a tablespoon of tamari or soy sauce for flavor.
- Sprinkle with sesame seeds and serve over cooked quinoa or brown rice.

This quick and nutritious stir-fry is packed with antioxidants, fiber, and essential nutrients.

MATCHA CHIA POPSICLES

- In a blender, combine 1 cup of coconut milk, 1 tablespoon of matcha powder, and 2 tablespoons of chia seeds.
- Blend until smooth and pour the mixture into popsicle molds.
- Freeze for a few hours until set.

Enjoy these refreshing and antioxidant-rich popsicles as a healthy treat that supports gut health and provides a natural energy boost.

With these recipe ideas, you can incorporate a variety of superfoods into your meals and snacks, making them not only delicious but also beneficial for your gut health and overall well-being.

Real-life Stories of Gut Health Transformation

Rachel's Triumph Over Digestive Struggles

Rachel had battled with severe digestive issues for as long as she could remember. The constant pain, bloating, and unpredictable bowel movements took a toll on her physical and emotional well-being.

Desperate for relief, she embarked on a journey to revitalize her gut health through the power of superfoods. With determination, Rachel incorporated fermented foods like sauerkraut and kombucha, as well as leafy greens and colorful vegetables into her daily meals.

Over time, she experienced a remarkable transformation. The pain subsided, the bloating diminished, and her digestion became regular and peaceful. Rachel's newfound digestive freedom brought tears of joy to her eyes as she finally regained control over her body and embraced a life of comfort and vitality.

Ethan's Liberation from Mental and Physical Struggles

Ethan had suffered silently from a combination of gut-related symptoms and mental health challenges. The constant fatigue, brain fog, and depressive episodes left him feeling trapped and disconnected from the world.

Determined to break free, Ethan embarked on a healing journey by embracing a diet rich in superfoods that nourish the gut and support mental well-being. He introduced probiotic-rich foods like yogurt and kefir, along with omega-3 fatty acid sources such as salmon and chia seeds.

The impact was profound. Ethan experienced a transformation like never before. His energy levels soared, his mind became clear and focused, and his mood stabilized. The weight of his struggles lifted, and Ethan finally felt liberated, embracing a life filled with hope, joy, and a newfound sense of purpose.